YOUR KNOWLEDGE HAS VALUE

- We will publish your bachelor's and master's thesis, essays and papers

- Your own eBook and book - sold worldwide in all relevant shops

- Earn money with each sale

Upload your text at www.GRIN.com and publish for free

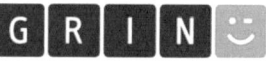

Bibliographic information published by the German National Library:

The German National Library lists this publication in the National Bibliography; detailed bibliographic data are available on the Internet at http://dnb.dnb.de .

This book is copyright material and must not be copied, reproduced, transferred, distributed, leased, licensed or publicly performed or used in any way except as specifically permitted in writing by the publishers, as allowed under the terms and conditions under which it was purchased or as strictly permitted by applicable copyright law. Any unauthorized distribution or use of this text may be a direct infringement of the author s and publisher s rights and those responsible may be liable in law accordingly.

Imprint:

Copyright © 2018 GRIN Verlag
Print and binding: Books on Demand GmbH, Norderstedt Germany
ISBN: 9783668648869

This book at GRIN:

https://www.grin.com/document/411951

Patrick Kimuyu

Approaches for Preventing Childhood Obesity

GRIN Verlag

GRIN - Your knowledge has value

Since its foundation in 1998, GRIN has specialized in publishing academic texts by students, college teachers and other academics as e-book and printed book. The website www.grin.com is an ideal platform for presenting term papers, final papers, scientific essays, dissertations and specialist books.

Visit us on the internet:

http://www.grin.com/

http://www.facebook.com/grincom

http://www.twitter.com/grin_com

Introduction

Over the past few decades, the burden of non-communicable diseases seems to have been increasing year-by-year. Childhood obesity serves as an outstanding example of non-communicable conditions whose consequences seem to have reached catastrophic levels. Evidence indicates that obesity and overweight trends have been increasing at alarming rates, especially over the past three decades [1]. This implies that the trends of obesity related health conditions are going to reflect upward changes in the future. According to Parsons, Power, Logan and Summerbell reaffirm that 70% of obese adults became obese during their childhood ages [2]. In retrospect, this phenomenon is believed to be attributable to the greater social inequality in developed countries as compared to developing countries [3]. Nevertheless, primary prevention strategies are required to reverse the diseases' trends across the world. Epidemiological rationale for the emphasis on primary prevention of childhood obesity is based on the fact that the condition is difficult to reverse with secondary interventions [4]. Therefore, this report is intended to inform the Federal Health Minister the scope of childhood obesity and the appropriate interventions which can address its impact.

Epidemiology of Childhood Obesity

Overall, epidemiological data from the World Health Organization indicate that over 40 million children aged below five years were obese or overweight by 2011 [5]. In Australia, it is reported that 25% of children are obese or overweight, whereas the adult population accounts for 60%. As such, the overall burden of obesity in Australia is estimated to be 7.5% [6]. Elsewhere in the United Kingdom, approximately 22.6% of children of preschool age are obese or overweight [7]. Similar trends have been reported in New Zealand where the population of obese children accounts for 31% of the total children population. A recent epidemiological survey indicated that the prevalence of childhood obesity had increased to 10% by 2012 from the rate of 8% recorded in 2006 [8]. Despite these differences in epidemiological trends of childhood obesity, it is apparent that its determinants are relatively the same in developed and developing countries.

Determinants of Childhood Obesity

The key determinants are physical inactivity, excess caloric intake, socio-economic status, socio-cultural factors, built environment, age, and gender. Of all these determinants, reduced physical activity and unhealthy dietary habits are considered be the main culprits for the raising prevalence trends of childhood obesity, worldwide [9]. As such, it is apparent that modifying these risk factors may reverse the prevalence of childhood obesity among the global population.

Proposed Approaches for the Prevention of Childhood Obesity

In this context, primary prevention approaches are deemed necessary for increasing physical activity, as well as adopting healthy dietary habits, rather than forcing obese individuals to lose weight [10]. Controlling weight gain for obese children, as well as secondary prevention of childhood obesity is also required to prevent the onset of obesity related conditions which reduce an individual's life expectancy and quality of life. In retrospect, it is apparent that there is no single preventive approach that has proven to reverse the prevalence of childhood obesity. However, some of the preventive approaches are known to be more effective than others. This implies that an integrated approach that combines several interventions may achieve appreciable success in combating the impact of childhood obesity across the globe. Therefore, this report recommends the adoption either or both of the proposed prevention strategies. The two main interventions which have been proven to reduce the prevalence of childhood obesity are school-based interventions and community-based interventions.

School-based Childhood Obesity Prevention Approach

In the past two decades, school-based interventions against childhood obesity have gained popularity. Different school-based preventive programs have been developed in different countries to prevent the increase of childhood obesity. Therefore, it is apparent that such approaches can help in addressing obesity epidemic in the country. In this context, a school-based obesity prevention approach should focus on reforming the curriculum to incorporate physical activity and integration of parents and teachers in obesity prevention programs.

The adoption of a structured learning curriculum which does not involve movement of children seems to be contributing to the increase of childhood obesity. According to Gardner, movement experiences are considered as some the main components of children's learning [11]. This is why the Institute of Medicine [IOM] observes that the pragmatic shift from movement-based learning to structured learning that focuses more on academic skills than physical activity may be contributing to the increasing prevalence of childhood obesity, especially in the United States, as well as other countries with a similar curriculum [12]. These concerns have been reaffirmed by Gehris, Gooze and Whitaker who investigated teachers' perception towards the role of movement in early childhood education programs. This qualitative survey indicated that movement experiences play integral roles in children's learning. For instance, this study revealed that movement is an innate need for children. Movement experiences were also found to augment children's success in school and life. Moreover, it was found out that movement experiences are essential in preparing children for learning. This is why teachers in this survey observed that a structured learning curriculum that excludes movement experiences as contradictory to the children's needs [13]. Therefore, the curriculum requires reforms to incorporate physical activity and nutritional education as the key elements of learning and obesity prevention among children.

In practice, engaging children in physical activity combined with healthier eating have proven to be an effective approach to prevent childhood obesity. The scientific rationale for integrating physical activity in childhood education is provided by two prospective studies which concluded that prudent diet and physical activity improves obesity related outcomes. Stone, McKenzie, Welk and Booth reviewed the impact of physical activity-oriented educational programs and concluded that a curriculum-based intervention is effective in improving children's health outcomes, especially with regard to obesity [14]. In another prospective study that involved school-based strategies including participation in physical education and sports, as well as healthier eating, the prevalence of obesity among 6th, 7th and 8th graders was found to decrease within two years. As a result, investigators in this study suggested policy-based changes at the education sector and school levels to promote physical activity through physical education and sports [15].

Moreover, the outcomes of two school-based programs; the Energize and APPLE (A Pilot Program for Lifestyle and Exercise) in New Zealand show how a curriculum-based approach can address the prevalence of childhood obesity epidemic in the country. The APPLE project focused on engaging children in non-curricular activities outside the classroom, as well as incorporating bursts of physical activity during classroom sessions. It also focused on promoting healthier dietary habits. Overall, the outcome of this intervention showed significant improvement of the key indicators of obesity. For instance, the mean BMI among the intervention group decreased by 0.26 points, whereas systolic blood pressure decreased by 4.8mmHg compared to the control group [16]. Similar outcomes were achieved in the Project Energize in which children in the participating schools recorded an average BMI reduction of 3% compared to that of the control children population [17].

However, the success of these programs showed that an effective school-based obesity prevention approach requires the integration of the key stakeholders, primarily parents and teachers. Middleton, Evans, Keegan, Bishop and Evans [18] describe teachers and parents as 'social agents' who play integral roles in enhancing the success of school-based healthy eating programs that are aimed at improving children's wellbeing including the prevention of childhood obesity.

Overall, the greatest strength of school-based obesity prevention programs is that the program can be designed to the targeted population. However, it is worth noting that parental influence serves as the key limitation [19].

Community-Based Childhood Obesity Prevention Approach

Community-based childhood obesity approach emerges as the second reliable intervention with the promise for reversing the current epidemiological trends of childhood obesity epidemic. An ideal community-based approach should focus on addressing food insecurity, modifying early life systems, promoting the development of healthy built environment, as well as discouraging unhealthy dietary intake. In retrospect, community-based childhood obesity interventions have gained popularity in developed countries. It is reported that such interventions hold immense promise for reducing the burden of childhood obesity [20]. In most cases, community-based childhood obesity prevention programs focus on modifying the key determinants of obesity [21].

Overall, a comprehensive community-based childhood obesity prevention program should target several elements. First, modification of early life systems should form the basis of such a program. It is suggested that modifying early life systems can bring the greatest impact in the prevention of obesity. This is so because the risks of obesity exhibit a carry-over effect, implying that obese conditions can be transitioned across an individual's developmental stages. As such, the key intervention targets are pregnancy, infancy and toddler stage. Intervention during pregnancy should focus on healthy weight gain and engagement in maternal care, whereas intervention during infancy should focus on breastfeeding, avoidance of screen time, support for healthy sleep behaviours and motor development. Finally, intervention during toddler years should focus on active play, healthy nutrition and limited screen time [22]. Ruel and Hoddinott emphasize on the provision of healthy nutrition in the early stages of development, in order to produce healthy adults [23]. Second, a comprehensive community-based childhood obesity prevention approach should focus on modifying eating habits of communities. This can be achieved through the introduction of measures which control nutrient intake and food-buying behaviour [24]. In this context, taxes on foods with high caloric or low nutritional value such as snacks and soft drinks have been found to be effective in controlling food-purchase behaviour, especially in the Canada and the US where such taxes have been implemented. It is also evident that food labelling can help people to choose healthy diets as it has been evidenced by the outcomes of the "Pick the Tick" program in New Zealand and Australia [25]. Finally, promoting the development of healthy built environment which supports physical activity can be a significant approach to the prevention of childhood obesity. This can be achieved through changes in urban planning to promote active modes of transport. For instance, safe cycling and walking routes should be designated, as well as implementing guidelines for building schools to ensure adequate playground is defined.

Overall, the strength of this approach is that is focuses on the ecological perspective [26]. On the other side, they have limited success due to issues related to their implementation. Ordinarily, such an approach requires the participation of the target communities and policy makers. As such, it may experience barriers in implementation as it has been the case with Obesity Prevention and Lifestyle (OPAL) program in South Australia [21].

Political Sensitivities to Proposed Interventions and Their Solution Mechanisms

Despite the benefits associated with these approaches, there are some political sensitivities that may arise from these proposals. Reforming the curriculum to incorporate movement experiences among children may be an uphill task. This is attributable to the fact that the education sector has shifted attention the promotion of academic skills due to the impact of global competitiveness. To solve this challenge, policy change can be addressed from the perspective of teachers who express willingness in engaging children in movement experiences. It is quite pleasing that teachers understand the role of movement in the child's learning and this is attributable to the emphasis provided by the main educational theories related to early childhood development [27].

On the other hand, the second approach which involves communities' behavioural changes and modification of built environment appears to involve policy-sensitive aspects. For instance, the introduction of taxes on foods and labelling bear immense political sensitivity. In a capitalism economy, such approaches may influence economic development of countries. However, this challenge can be addressed through the implementation of a multi-sectoral approach which is incentive-based. For instance, food manufacturers can be given incentives which promote the production of healthy foods.

Conclusion

Conclusively, it is apparent that the consequences of obesity epidemic are catastrophic. Therefore, there is an urgent need for federal-based prevention approaches which hold the promise for reducing the prevalence of childhood obesity. Therefore, the proposed prevention approaches appears appropriate for promoting healthy living and quality of life.

References

1 Wang Y, Lobstein T. Worldwide trends in childhood overweight and obesity. Int J Pediatr Obes. 2006 May; 1(1):11-25.

2 Parsons TJ, Power C, Logan S, Summerbell CD. Childhood predictors of adult obesity: a systematic review. Int J Obes Relat Metab Disord. 1999 Nov; 23(8):S1-107.

3 Monteiro CA, Conde WL, Lu B, Popkin BM. Obesity and inequities in health in the developing world. Int J Obes Relat Metab Disord. 2004 Oct; 28:1181–6.

4 Oude Luttikhuis H, Baur L, Jansen H, Shrewsbury VA, O'Malley C, Stolk RP, Summerbell CD. Interventions for treating obesity in children. Cochrane Database Syst Rev.2009 Sep;1: CD001872.

5 Redsell SA, Edmonds B, Swift JA, Siriwardena AN, Weng S, Nathan D, Glazebrook C. Systematic review of randomised controlled trials of interventions that aim to reduce the risk, either directly or indirectly, of overweight and obesity in infancy and early childhood. Maternal and Child Nutrition, 2016 Jan; 12: 24 – 38.

6 Clark R, Armstrong R, Waters E. Local government and obesity prevention: An evidence resource. Interventions to prevent obesity in early year's settings; tackling food insecurity and built environment changes to support physical activity. Geelong: CO-OPS Secretariat, Deakin University; 2010.

7 Health and Social Care Information Centre. National Child Measurement Programme: England, 2012/2013 [Internet]. [Cited 2017 Dec 25]. Available from: http://www.hscic.gov.uk/catalogue/PUB13115/nati-chil-meas-prog-eng-2012-2013-rep.pdf

8 Mulrine H. Interventions to prevent childhood obesity Literature review. Christchurch: Canterbury District Health Board; 2013.

9 Kar, SS, Dube R, Kar SS. Childhood obesity-an insight into preventive strategies. Avicenna J Med. 2014 Oct-Dec; 4(4): 88–93.

10 Caterson ID, Gill TP. Obesity: epidemiology and possible prevention. Best Pract Res Clin Endocrinol Metab. 2002 Dec; 16(4):595-610.

11 Gardner H. Frames of mind: the theory of multiple intelligences. New York: Basic Books; 2011.

12 Institute of Medicine. Early childhood obesity prevention policies. Washington DC: National Academies Press; 2011.

13 Gehris JS, Gooze RA, Whitaker RC. Teachers' perceptions about children's movement and learning in early childhood education programmes. Child: care, health and development, 2014 Jan; 41(1): 122–131.

14 Stone EJ, McKenzie TL, Welk GJ, Booth ML. Effects of physical activity interventions in youth. Review and synthesis. Am J Prev Med. 1998 Nov; 15:298–315.

15 Dwyer T, Coonan WE, Leitch DR, Hetzel BS, Baghurst RA. An investigation of the effects of daily physical activity on the health of primary school students in South Australia. Int J Epidemiol. 1983 Sep; 12:308–313.

16 Taylor RW, McAuley KA, Barbezat W, Farmer VL, Williams SM, Mann JI. Two-year follow-up of an obesity prevention initiative in children: the APPLE project. Am J Clin Nutr. 2008 Nov; 88(5): 1371-1377.

17 Rush E, Reed P, McLennan S, Coppinger T, Simmons D, Graham D. A school-based obesity control programme: Project Energize. Two-year outcomes. Br J Nutr. 2012 Feb; 107(4): 581-587.

18 Middleton G, Evans AB, Keegan RJ, Bishop D, Evans D. The importance of parents and teachers as stakeholders in school-based healthy eating programs [Internet]. [Cited

2017 Dec 20]. Available from:

http://eprints.lincoln.ac.uk/11965/1/Middleton%20et%20al.%202013_PreprintNOVA _doc.pdf

19 Ickes MJ, McMullen J, Haider T, Sharma M. Global school-based childhood obesity interventions: a review. Int J Environ Res Public Health, 2014 Sep; 11(9): 8940–8961.

20 Swinburn BA, Sacks G, Hall KD, McPherson K, Finegood DT, Moodie ML, Gortmaker SL. The global obesity pandemic: shaped by global drivers and local environments. Lancet, 2011 Aug; 378: 804–14.

21 Richards Z, Kostadinov I, Jones M, Richard L, Cargo M. Assessing implementation fidelity and adaptation in a community-based childhood obesity prevention intervention. Health Education Research, 2014 Sep; 2014: 1-15.

22 Nader PR, Huang T, Gahagan S, Kumanyika S, Hammond RA, Christoffel KK. Next steps in obesity prevention: altering early life systems to support healthy parents, infants, and toddlers. Childhood Obesity, 2012 Jun; 8(3): 195-204.

23 Ruel M, Hoddinott J. Investing in early childhood nutrition. Washington DC: IFPRI; 2008.

24 Guo X, Popkin BM, Mroz TA, Zhai F. Food price policy can favorably alter macronutrient intake in China. J Nutr. 1999 Sep; 129:994–1001.

25 Young L, Swinburn B. Impact of the Pick the Tick food information programme on the salt content of food in New Zealand. Health Promot Int. 2002 Aug; 17:13–19.

26 Ickes MJ, Sharma M. A systematic review of community-based childhood obesity prevention programs. Journal of Obesity & Weight Loss Therapy, 2013 Aug; 3:188.

27 Hohmann M, Weikart DP. Educating young children: active learning practices for preschool and child care programs. Ypsilanti: High/Scope Press; 1995.

YOUR KNOWLEDGE HAS VALUE

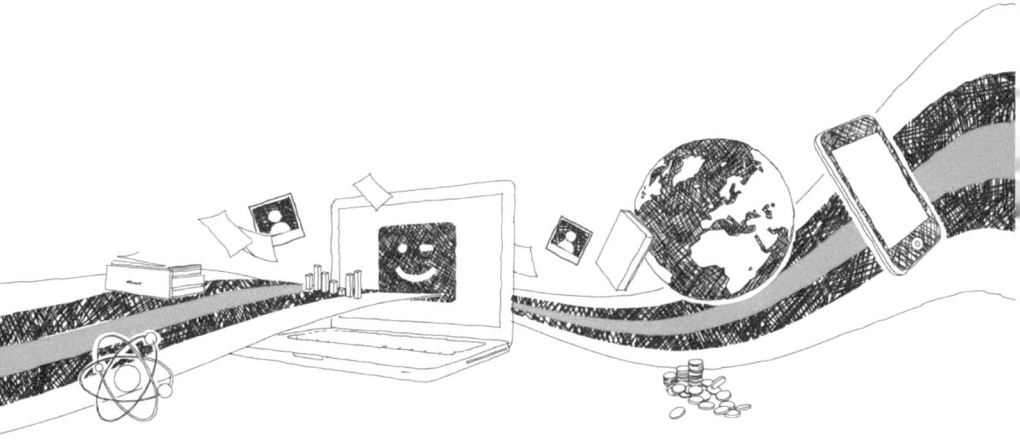

- We will publish your bachelor's and master's thesis, essays and papers

- Your own eBook and book - sold worldwide in all relevant shops

- Earn money with each sale

Upload your text at www.GRIN.com
and publish for free